A GUIDE
to
HEALTHY LIVING

A GUIDE
to
HEALTHY LIVING
SAFE WEIGHT LOSS
at
LITTLE OR NO COST

---

by

Apollone S. Reid

Edited by
The Late Dr. Lorna Nembhard
Dr. Prudencia Kintaudi

Part I—Copyright 1997—Jamaica W.I.

This book was printed in the United States of America.

To order additional copies of this book, contact:
Xlibris Corporation
1-888-795-4274
www.Xlibris.com
Orders@Xlibris.com
58550

ACKNOWLEDGEMENT

I would like to express thanks to Almighty God who has strengthened me to endure and triumph over the turbulent experiences of ill health. This has led to an increase in my understanding and wisdom. In a miraculous way, He provided the environment and the opportunity for me to gain knowledge.

To the patients attending my physical therapy clinic who encouraged me to write this instructive piece, please know that without your insistence, this would still be only a concept.

I am eternally thankful to the late Dr. Lorna Nembhard who encouraged me constantly when she herself needed encouragement through difficult times and whose editorial assistance has been invaluable. Her sudden and untimely passing caused me to shelf this project for many years. I now feel that reviving this work will no doubt positively impact public health, thus contributing to a healthier, more productive nation.

I am so indebted to Dr. Prudencia Kintaudi for the fantastic work done in reviving the spirit of this book. I am at a loss for appropriate words to express my gratitude for the editing done by Dr. Kintaudi and the retyping of Part 1 done by her assistant Erica Arrendondo, in order to facilitate its publication at such short notice. I am forever grateful.

EDITORIAL COMMENTS

In a world where the majority of individuals are focused on "quick-fixes" and achieving success by the pursuit of fame, fortune and professional success, not many take the time to address the issue of health, including the necessary ingredients of life management which will ensure that they will live healthy lives long enough to enjoy the successes that they have achieved.

My hat is off to Apollone Reid who has presented the issues of weight loss and achieving a healthy life-style in realistic ways that everyone can understand. She has taken time, during her own pursuits of "life . . . liberty . . . (and) happiness" to write about the things that matter, but are most often forgotten.

I was inspired by the logical activities and diets that were proposed and admired the fact that various substitutes and options were offered, which would fit various life-styles and cultures.

This book became the catalyst that jolted me from an existence of complacency and a life that was dedicated to the pursuits of my happiness—a life of full-time dedication to the sedentary activities of professional and educational development, to one that seeks a more balanced "life-enabling" approach.

I know that this book will be inspiring to those who choose to carve a few minutes of their time out in order to read this book, and realize that it is time to take action and take control of our lives.

Apollone Reid lives what she preaches: she follows her own advice—she lives a healthy life style, and exercises regularly. As I looked at her and saw the embodiment of a vibrant, healthy individual, I made the critical decision to carve a few minutes out of my life and take the challenge to stand on her proverbial shoulders and become more than I have chosen to be.

MY MESSAGE TO ALL WHO LOOK AT THIS BOOK IS: TAKE THE CHALLENGE AND BE THE VIBRANT HEALTHY INDIVIDUAL YOU WERE DESIGNED TO BE.

Prudencia Kintaudi, M.D.
(Editor)

DEDICATION

This book is dedicated to the many patients who have attended my physical therapy practice and who have been unable to find medical answers to their physical pain. Also to those who have fought the endless "battle of the bulges."

I wish to express my gratitude to my husband, Juan, who allowed me to put prime time into the writing of this book, and to my children Ryan, Juanita, and Patrice, who I hope will use the instructions in this book to assist in maintaining good health. Thanks also to my mother, Joyce Peterkin, without whose help, I would not have been able to carve out the time necessary from my busy schedule, to live a physically active and balanced lifestyle. My greatest desire is also for my granddaughters, Emma and Eden to realize the benefits of using the instructions in this book. I dedicate this work to the aforementioned.

To the people of the world, I dedicate this to you, with hearty wishes that each of you will become stronger, because you have become healthier from having read this book, and subsequently are making the lifestyle adjustments necessary for ultimately gaining long, happy, and purposeful existence.

TABLE OF CONTENTS

INTRODUCTION

Much has been written recently about healthy lifestyles, safe weight loss and dieting. Most of the programs designed have proven to be too costly to maintain and involve stringent guidelines that place too much burden on the individual to adhere to. Moreover, once broken result in the individual reverting to the old way of eating and living, return of weight and the practice of unhealthy lifestyle.

This program is designed to give you an understanding of the life long benefits of healthy living and the way you can incorporate it into your daily lifestyle at little or no additional cost. All it takes is some minor adjustments in the way you eat and organize your daily activities. It is hoped that a responsibility to self will be instilled in every reader as the reality of the distinct connections between nutrition, exercise and chronic, non-communicable diseases are realized.

The aim is to prevent the negative effects seen after fad diets and costly health programs have ended and so eliminate the yo-yo effects of weight loss and weight gain. These simple changes are easily adopted into becoming a natural practice in the way we live and move and have our being. Thus this program eventually becomes no cost to us as this will be the normal way of shopping, cooking, eating, functioning, and playing.

In the past, it was acceptable to believe that human beings inherited certain diseases from their fore parents and despite how we changed our eating habits and the way we lived; we doomed to suffer the same diseases that plagued them. It was generally accepted also that if one came from an obese family line, one had to be obese.

FAD DIETS

ON DIET

OFF DIET

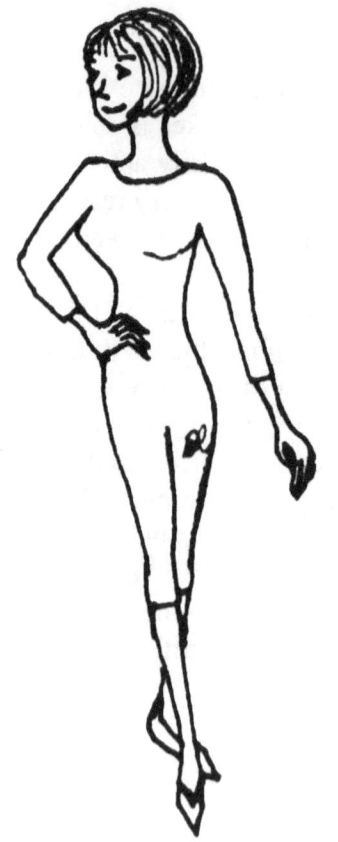

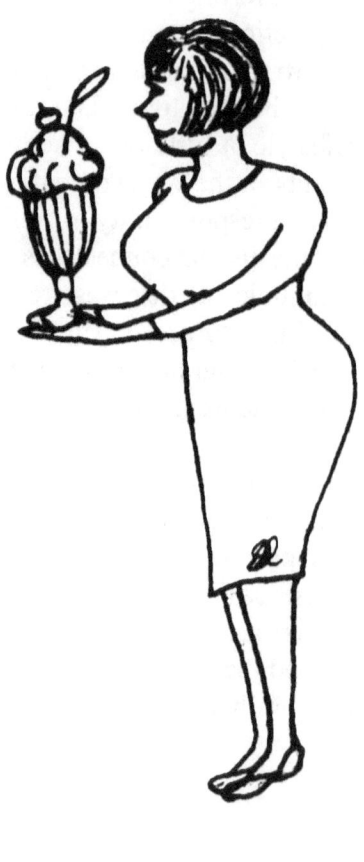

All throughout my life I had to listen to persons declare the doom of obesity on me, simply because I possessed a bone structure which some persons know as a large skeletal frame. The derogatory tones of these declarations made me determine at age ten years that these persons would never live to see these predictions over my life come true. So, on entering boarding school at ten years, I decided to make every effort to be chosen for the school tennis team which would enable me to play for one hour, five days per week. Although it was difficult to eat healthy, mainly from a lack of knowledge on the importance of nutrition, I noticed that regular exercises affected my health in a positive way. I never suffered from menstrual cramps at school, like the girls who avoided exercises did. However, during the holidays, when I did not have the facilities to play tennis, I experienced a moderate amount of cramps and menorrahgia. I also noticed that I packed on weight whenever I did not do regular exercises for any extended period of my life.

As age progressed, I suffered from many health problems associated with consistent constipation, soft tissue and skeletal pain, anxiety, decreased energy and allergies. I participated in many weight loss programs, fad diets and pill popping health programs which demanded so much discipline and discomfort that I could never enjoy life while I was on them and eagerly looked forward to the termination of the programs when I could again eat the food I had come to love. Although I lost weight each time, I regained weight in less time than it took to lose it. In addition, I also seemed to put on some bonus pounds. I had to make an effort to eat less than I had been eating before going on each diet program. In three days of dieting, my five feet, four inches frame had moved from an attractive one hundred and twenty eight pound form to a round middle aged look, sporting one hundred and fifty pounds, accompanied by constant aches and pains.

Desperate to find a cure for the pains, I visited a nutritionist who put me on a three day cleansing program. Though I was only able to tolerate this for two days, the intensity of the pain was reduced by sixty to seventy percent.

GOOD NUTRITION
EXERCISE
GOOD HABITS

SATISFACTORY

EXISTENCE

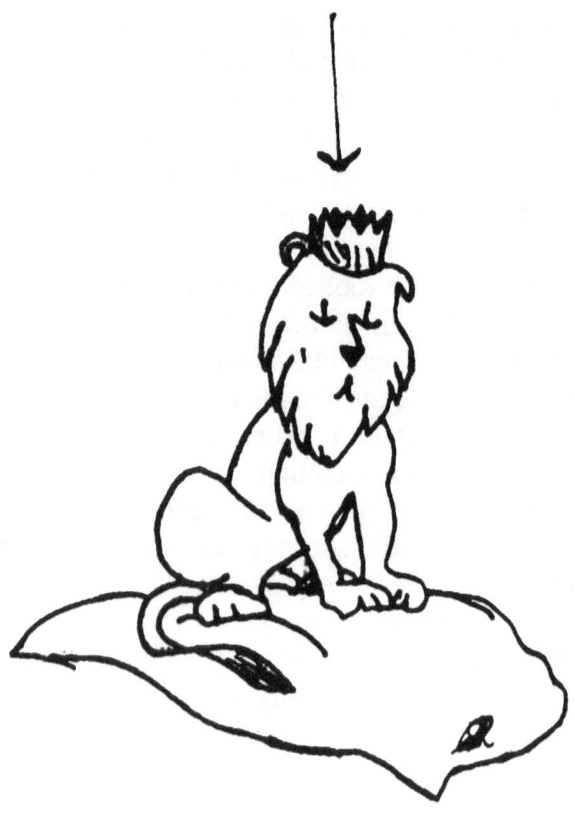

As I sat in her office and listened to her tapes on how to eat in the mornings, I noted that she actually suggested some of the very things I had been using recently which afforded me some amount of relief at times. A couple of weeks after going through her cleansing program, I discovered that the pains were again increasing in intensity. The masters I public health program that I was reading for had just completed its nutrition section. With this new knowledge and my experience with cleansing, I worked out a new program of eating and exercising for myself. Within three months, I had lost fifteen pounds by increasing my starch, vegetable and fruit intake and decreasing my meat and dairy products intake. I exercised three to four times per week and tried to walk to classes instead of driving the less than quarter of a mile. Today, a mother of three, at age forty three, I weigh one hundred and thirty five pounds and have twice the energy I had before, changing my lifestyle and none of the pain.

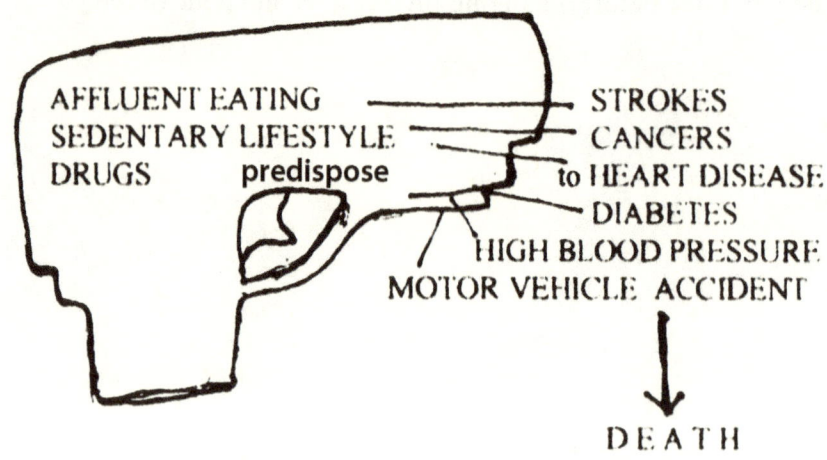

AFFLUENT EATING — STROKES
SEDENTARY LIFESTYLE — CANCERS
DRUGS   predispose   to HEART DISEASE
— DIABETES
HIGH BLOOD PRESSURE
MOTOR VEHICLE ACCIDENT

DEATH

CHAPTER 1

UNDERSTANDING DISEASE AND NUTRITION

This chapter highlights important points from lectures given to master of public health students in the department of social and preventive medicine, University of West Indies, Mona campus, in 1996.

With the advent of immunization, improved sanitation and portable water, there has been a decrease in the prevalence of infectious diseases and their contribution to mortality. In our society today, the major causes of and contributors to death are cancers, strokes, heart diseases, and high blood pressure, diabetes, and motor vehicle accidents. Sinha (1995) stated that one of every two to four deaths is now due to these non-communicable chronic diseases.

Some effects of these diseases

Sinha (1995) made the following associations:

DIABETICS have— four times more heart disease than persons without the disease.

Six times more strokes.

DIABETES is— the number one cause of blindness.

responsible for forty five percent of all leg and foot amputations.

Responsible for ten percent of serious kidney disease.

EFFECTS OF STROKE

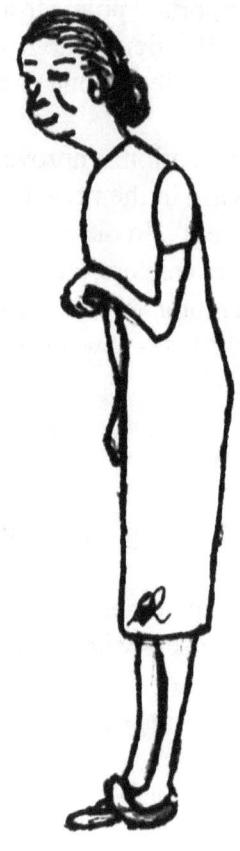

HEART DISEASE— Seventy five percent of the people who get heart attacks die suddenly or before reaching hospital or during their hospitalization.

CANCERS— One of the leading causes of premature deaths in the Caribbean today.

STROKES— Twenty three percent of persons with strokes die within one week of having suffered the stroke.

Another 23 percent die within one year

Of those who survive, only 20 percent are able to go back to work.

Many stroke victims develop abnormal patterns in the affected limbs which become disabled and non-functional. This often is the result of lack of immediate and appropriate physical therapy designed to inhibit these abnormal patterns associated with strokes.

OBESITY— Fat persons have higher than normal rates of premature deaths

THINKING HEALTHY

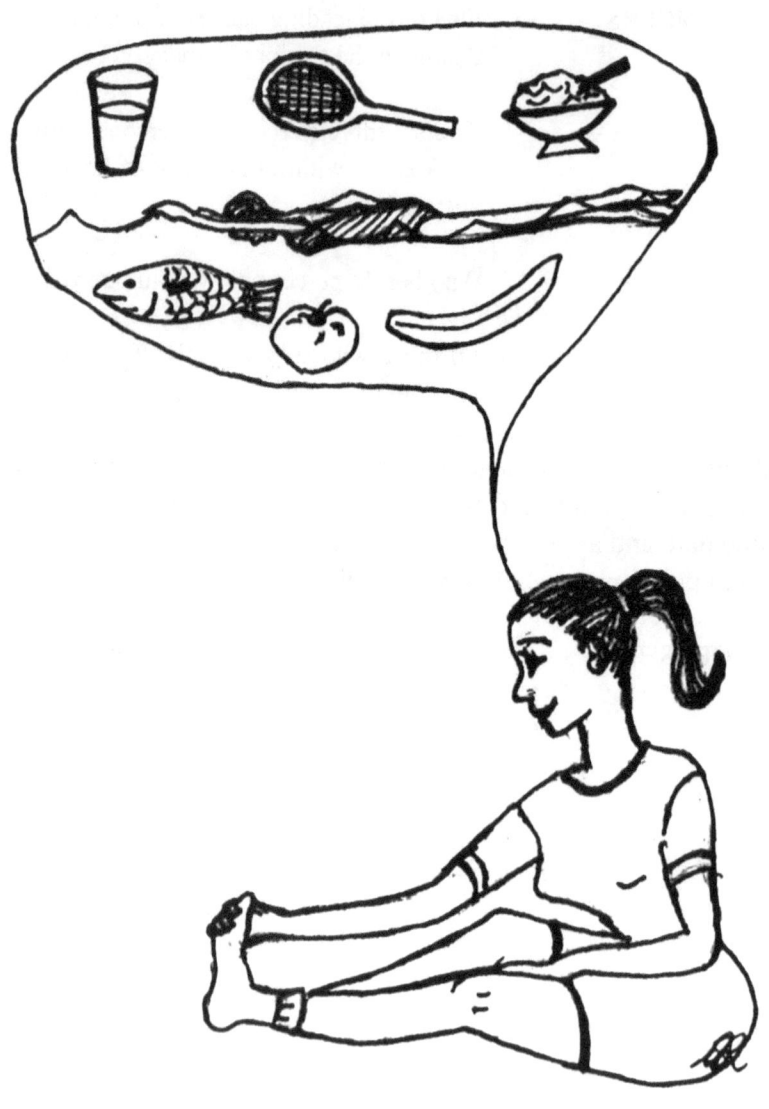

Persons who are twenty percent overweight have twice the chance of getting diabetes. (This weight keeps doubling for every twenty percent weight gain).

Fat persons have three to six times higher rates of high blood pressure.

Persons who are five to fifteen percent overweight have deaths from heart attacks twice as often.

For those twenty five percent or more overweight, the number of heart attacks is five times higher than normal.

Overweight men have higher mortality ratio for colo-rectal and prostate cancer, while overweight women have higher ratios for cancer of the uterus, gallbladder, cervix, ovary, breast, and also have a higher ratio of gout and arthritis than normal.

- The Centers for Disease Control and Prevention, (CDC) (2009) concurs with the above findings, stating that more than one-third of U.S. adults (more than 72 million people) and 16% of U.S. children are obese. This increases the risk for the development of Diabetes and heart disease in both the children and the adults. The CDC has the leading cause of death in the U.S. as heart disease, and the second leading cause of death as cancers. The CDC also emphasized concern regarding strokes, being the third leading cause of death in the U.S., and resulting in over 143,579 people dying each year in the United States. It named strokes as the leading cause of serious long-term disability, having approximately 795,000 cases occurring in the U.S. each year.

A recent U. S. Surgeon General's (2009) report summarized Sinnha's (2005) findings as it noted that obesity is an epidemic and is responsible for more than 300,000 deaths annually in the U.S. Since these facts

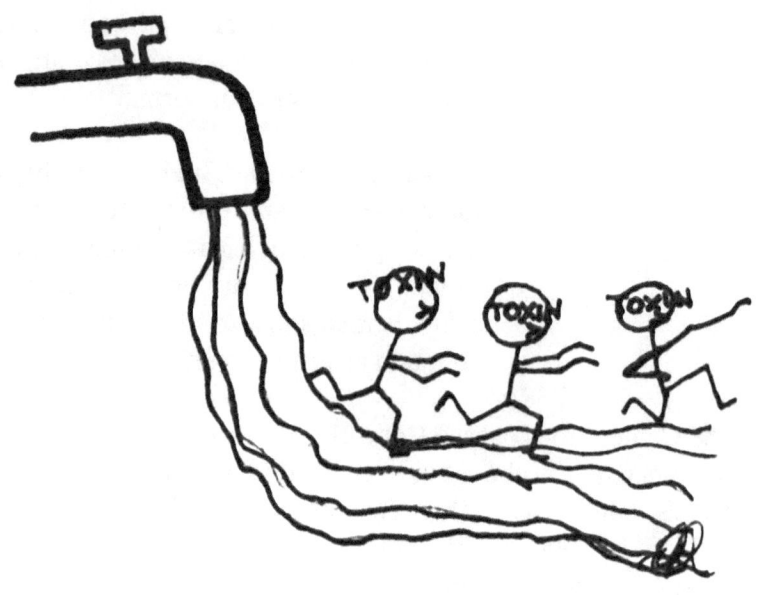

are known, it is vital for us to change our patterns of thinking and the reinforcements we put in our youth. Remember, it is not what we eat today that affects us, but what we have been eating over the years of growing up and maturing. Obesity must therefore cease to be seen as a sign of prosperity as in fact it is a slow killer. According to the 1983 Metropolitan Life Insurance Company Height and Weight table for women, a woman is considered obese if she is twenty percent over her ideal weight. Thus, if she is five feet tall and of small frame, her ideal weight is between 106 and 118 pounds. If she is between 126 and 141 pounds, then she is twenty percent over her ideal weight.

In essence, obesity is a form of malnourishment or bad nourishment, and usually results from excess intake of energy rich foods like sugar based products, fats, oils, gravies, fried foods, ice cream, alcoholic beverages, etc. These eventually make you unhealthy, creating medical expenses which eventually contribute to the economic burden of the nation.

Staying healthy

The best way to stay healthy is to avoid complications. Regular exercises, healthy eating, drinking lots of water daily and keeping the body free of drugs, are the best ways of staying healthy.

Exercise

Persons who exercise regularly will benefit through reduced obesity, improved heart function, increased circulation and thus improved resistance to diseases. Sinha (1995) attributed the following to regular exercises:

- 50% decreased chance of getting heart disease than persons who are inactive
- Up to 50% chance of getting high blood pressure. Blood pressure can be reduced by approximately 10mmHg with regular exercises.
- Associated with preventing non-insulin dependent diabetes.
- Lowers the risk of many cancers
- Prevents age related thinning of bones (osteoporosis)
- Diminishes physical and functional changes associated with aging

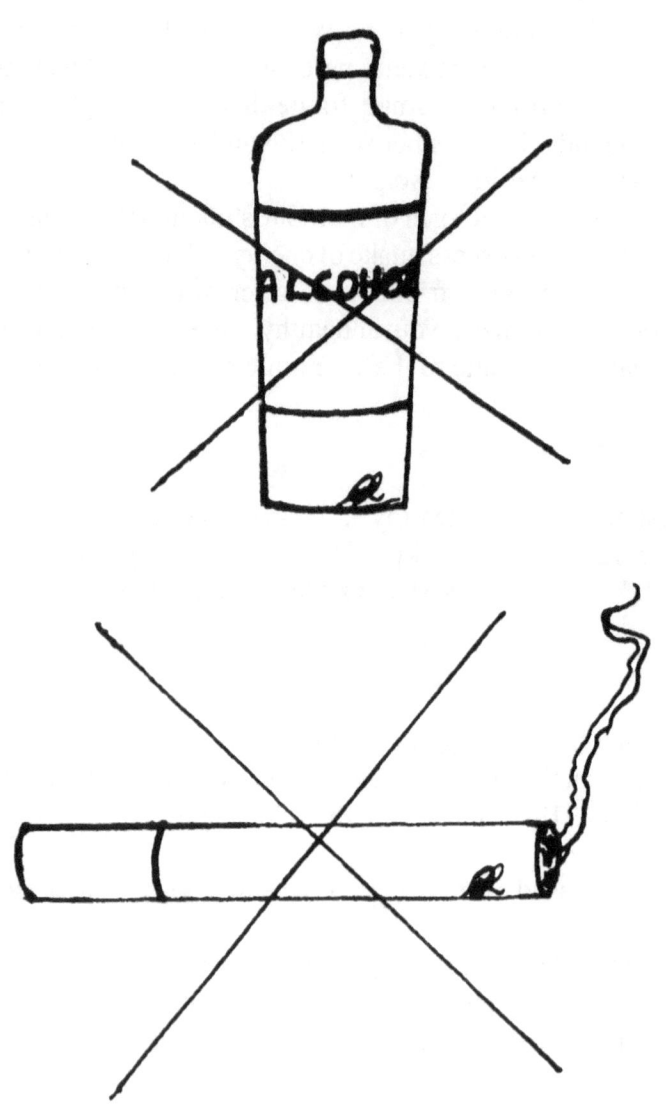

Regular exercises do not have to be long and strenuous. Twenty or more minutes of active exercise done four or more times per week will prove quite adequate.

Other Factors

Besides eating healthy and exercising regularly, we must keep out bodies free of drugs such as cigarettes and alcohol. Highlights of the 1996 epidemiology lectures to master of public health (MPH) students included the recognition that ninety percent of all lung cancer cases are smokers. Also that smoking has been implicated in heart diseases, vascular diseases, stomach ulcers, strokes, hemorrhaging in pregnancy, premature deliveries, small birth weight babies, spontaneous deliveries, chest conditions such as chronic bronchitis, emphysema and many more. The Cleveland Clinic (2009) reported that smoking is a major cause of atherosclerosis, thickening the walls of the arteries and blocking blood flow through the arteries, which may eventually lead to a heart attack.

Alcohol has been implicated in cirrhosis of the liver, diseases of the pancreas and stomach, cancers of the throat, larynx, stomach and motor vehicle accidents.

Fats and Cancers

The following synopsis of some lectures to 1996 MPH students will help to show the relationship between dietary fats, heart disease, and cancers:

It is believed that fats high in low density lipoproteins and low in high density lipoproteins are not promoters of cancers as those containing linoleic acids. These, however, are believed to increase cholesterol level thus hardening the arteries and predisposing heart diseases and strokes.

Those rich in oleic acids, that have a high level of high density lipoprotein and a low level of low density lipoprotein are thought to promote cancers.

Oils with a balance of both high and low density lipoproteins are now thought to be safer. One such oil is coconut oil, once thought to be dangerous as it is saturated.

LIFTING

INCORRECT

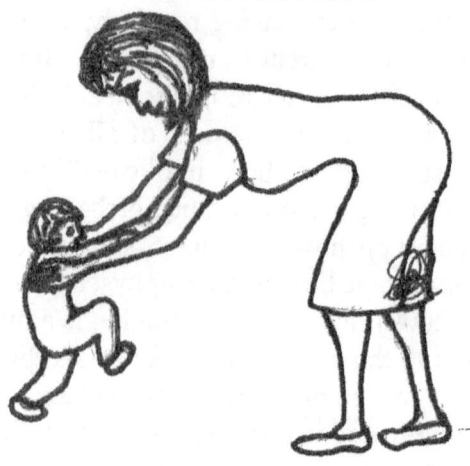

CORRECT

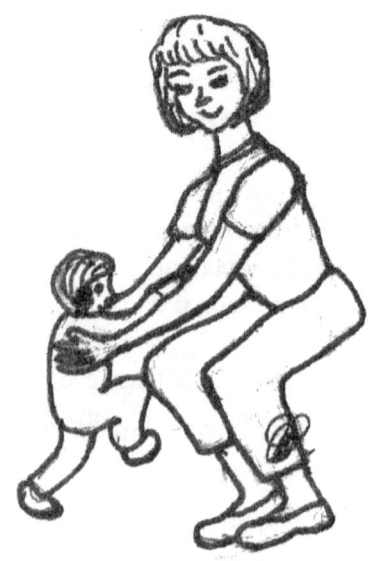

However, because it is a vegetable oil and because of its chemical make up, it is felt to be one of the safer oils to use. We must however be careful to note that studies on this are still incomplete.

Cleveland Clinic (2009) recommends that saturated fats should be avoided since they are linked to heart disease. They can be found in regular cheese, regular margarine, regular ice cream, skin of chicken. The Cleveland Clinic also recommends avoiding foods rich trans-fats such as cookies, crackers, cakes, French fries, onion rings, and donuts.

Other Foods

Epidemiology lectures to master of public health students also highlighted and recommended diets rich in fiber which have been correlated with lower risk of colon cancers. The lectures noted that vitamin A and carotenoids protect against many cancers. These elements were noted to be found in fish, liver, egg yolk, cheese, callaloo, carrots, pumpkin, mango, and papaya.

Other Aids

We should not forget the role of proper body mechanics in preventing injury to the musculoskeletal system of our body. The way we sit, stand, lift articles, bend to pick up items and carry out functions of daily living, plays an important role in the preservation of our musculoskeletal system.

Abuse of this system through improper function inevitably results in painful signs and symptoms which may be functionally disabling.

Twenty minutes a day
Energizes while you play
Four days a week
Health is what you seek

CHAPTER 2

REGULATING EXERCISES

The importance of regular exercises cannot be overemphasized. However, exercises must be properly regulated to suit the individual and his or her condition.

A healthy person who has never done active exercise should start out slowly, with short sessions. This will prevent overexertion which may lead to de-motivation.

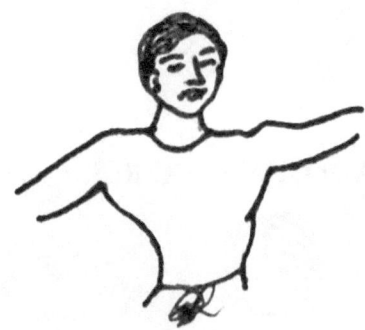

Initial ten minute sessions of uninterrupted jogging, lawn tennis, swimming or other dynamic activity may be increased by three to five minutes each successive day, with individuals tuning into their own bodies. If breathing becomes difficult of does not return to the effortless state within two to three minutes, the individual should consult his physician.

Persons suffering from any illness should exercise initially under the direct supervision of a medical practitioner, nurse or therapist experienced in the area of exercise physiology as it relates to the different medical conditions.

Exercises are effective when done at least four times per week, lasting more than twenty minutes per session.

TOO MUCH EXERCISE

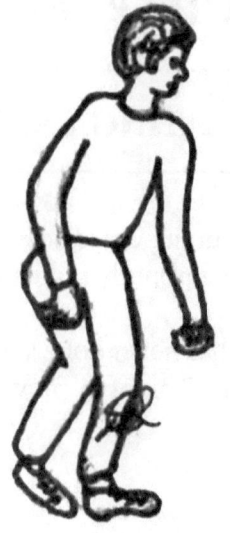

ADEQUATE EXERCISE

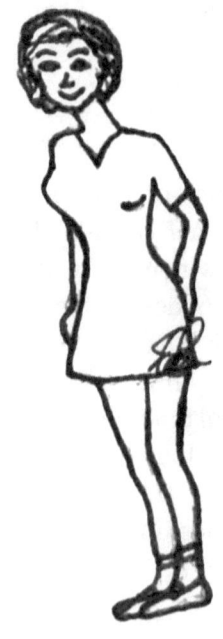

Exercises should be an ongoing activity and not seasonal. You will only benefit now from exercises being done at this time of your life. Many persons like to speak about the fact that they used to be very active when they were young. This will not be of much benefit to them now that they are old as this is not an old aged pension you can invest in during youthful days in cash in during old age.

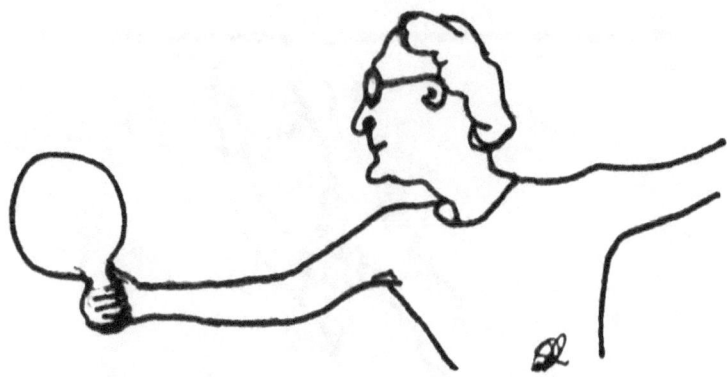

One benefit of exercise is increased circulation. If the circulation is increased, it means nutrients that the body needs to function efficiently can be more adequately transported around the body.

Another benefit of exercise is prevention of backaches and neck and shoulder pain. When exercising under stressful conditions, the muscles tend to become tight or go into spasm. This is especially apparent in the muscles around the neck and shoulders. Simple neck rolling and stretching for one minute every hour will help release the spasms or tension in the muscles and thus prevent pain.

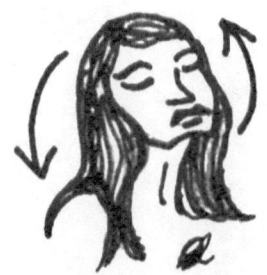

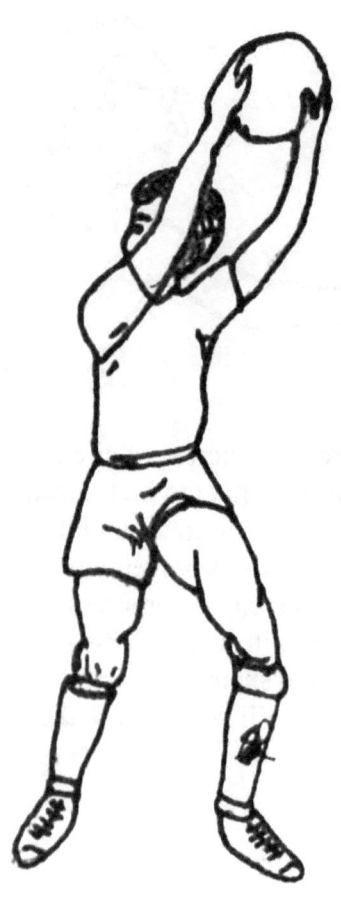

Prolonged static postures can put strain on the muscles of the low back thus causing low back pain and ultimate weakening of the area. This may result in inadequate support of the spine and functionally mal-aligned postures. Simple stretching exercises done lying on the back and holding the knees into the chest will help relieve low back tension.

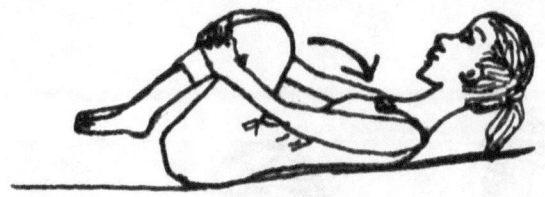

Lying on the belly, with arms by the side, while lifting the head and shoulders up, holding for five seconds each, will help to strengthen the extensors of the back. This will assist in supporting the spine and keeping it in proper alignment.

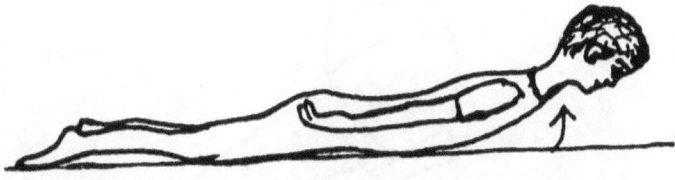

The role of the abdominal muscles in supporting the spine must not be forgotten. Lying on the back with knees bent and hands stretched over the knees as the head and shoulders are lifted up off the floor will strengthen the abdominals. The chin should be tucked into the chest and each lift held for five

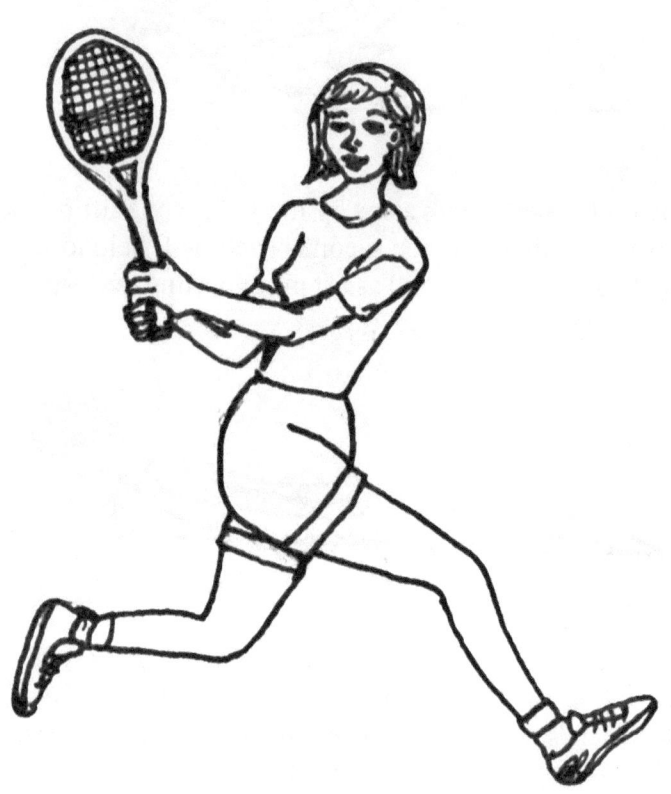

seconds. The shoulders do not need to be raised more than four inches off the floor.

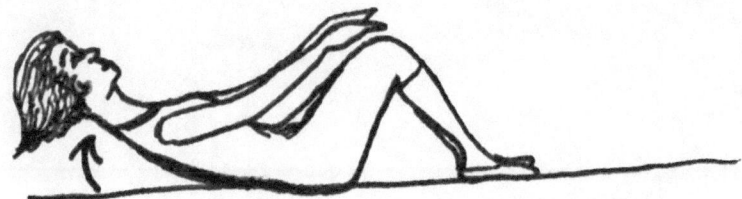

For maximum effectiveness, each exercise should be done ten times, every morning and evening. The most convenient times for most persons have been just after getting out of bed in the mornings and just before going to bed at nights.

Let's watch the food we eat
Avoid too much meat
Sugars, fats and sweets
That's not too big a feat

CHAPTER 3

EATING TO STAY HEALTHY

Two decades ago, it was impressed on us that we should eat lots of meats, very little starchy foods, lots of vegetables and fruits. Many of us have experimented with this combination but have not found the answer in this formula for maintaining our energy, weight loss or for staying healthy. Besides, many who have tried to lose weight by this formula have reported constant feeling of hunger or dissatisfaction, low energy level and immediate weight gain on ceasing to use this method.

Eating healthy must be a way of life. I found out that the most practical and easy to maintain diet was one in which sweet drinks were eliminated. Many persons complain about the bland taste of water as an excuse for not wanting to give up sweet drinks. When we drink that, there is no real cure for diabetes and it inevitably leads to premature death, this should be some impetus for at least wanting to try eliminating sweet dreams from our diet. The body needs to be cleansed of toxins daily. What better way to do it than to drink six to eight ounce glasses of water each day. The difficulty with most persons is starting. Once a logical rational approach is taken, then drinking water becomes a pleasure. Many persons who used to think it was impossible to drink water, now report that once they started they never had the desire to revert to drinking sweet drinks. The body needs fluids and not sugars. Moreover, the body obtains its supply of sugar from so many of the other vital foods that it takes in. Complex starches from staples such as ground provisions are broken down into sugar. Our fruits have an abundant supply of sugar.

BALANCED DIET

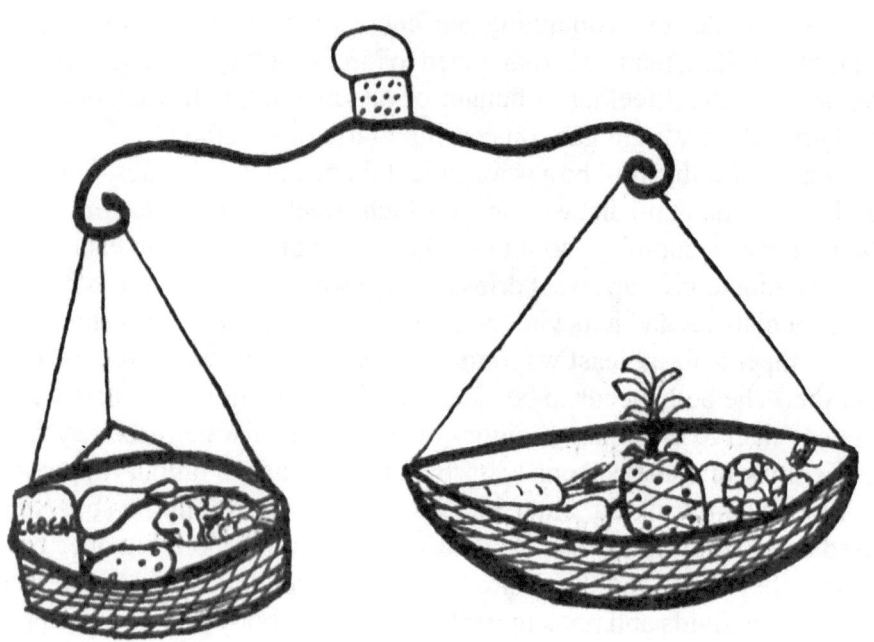

Drinking adequate amounts of water daily will improve your bowel activity and enhance the functioning of many vital body organs. Fluid intake may also be complemented with natural unsweetened fruit juices without preservatives.

I have found that persons who suffered gross constipation got relief after drinking one glass of warm lime water (1 lime) followed by eating a large ripe banana. This had to be done first thing after awaking each morning. Bowel activity could be enhanced also by eating a bowl of unsweetened oat cereal, having been cooked for approximately one minute.

Our food intake is important. Foods are categorized in groups and will be most beneficial to us when taken in the correct proportions. The basic four food groups eaten daily should be in the ratio 4:2:1:1 for staples, peas and beans, vegetables, foods from animals (Sinha, 1995). Staples include cereals, starchy fruits, roots and tubers. Sinha recommends the following amounts of each food group for adults and older children in the Caribbean daily:

12-18 ounces (340-500g)	ground provisions
6-9 ounces (170-250g)	cereals
2-3 ounces (60-90g)	legumes and nuts
4-6 ounces (120-170g)	food from animals
1 ¾-2 ½ lbs (800-1200g)	fruits and vegetables
1-1 ½ ounces (30-50g)	fats and oils
1 ½ ounces (50g)	sugars

Some food classification

Ground Provisions—breadfruit, dasheen, malanga, cassava, yucca, green bananas, potato, sweet potato, pumpkin, yam, plantain. These food items have similar nutrients, one being able to be a substitute for the other.

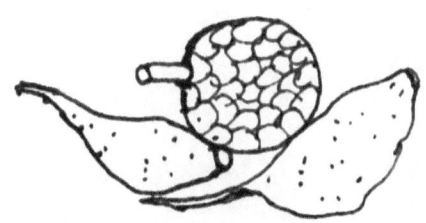

ENERGIZED

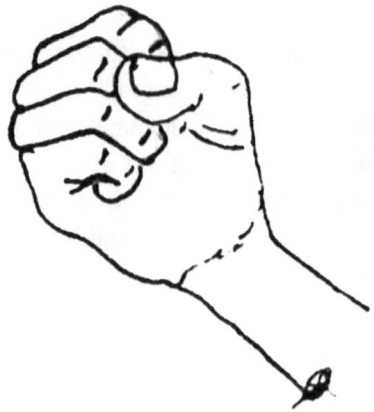

Cereals—   flour, bread, corn, oats, cornmeal, rice.

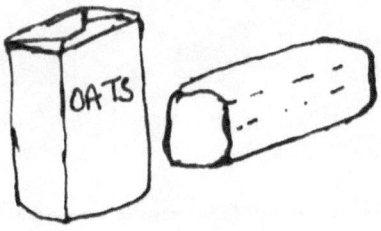

Fruits and Vegetables— pineapple, oranges, sweetsop, sour sop, watermelon, ripe banana, mango, naseberry, apples, carrot, tomatoes, lettuce, cabbage, green pepper, okra, callalloo.

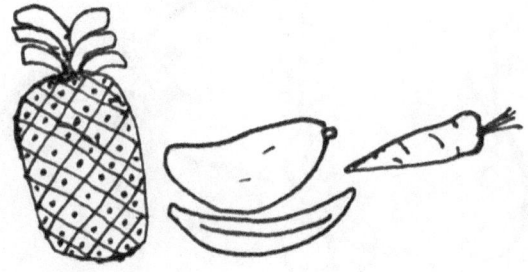

Food from Animals—   milk, cheese, eggs, fish, chicken.

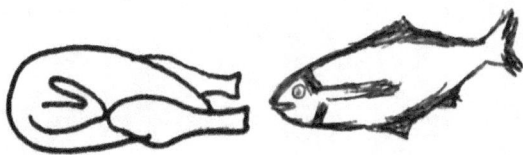

FIRST INTAKE

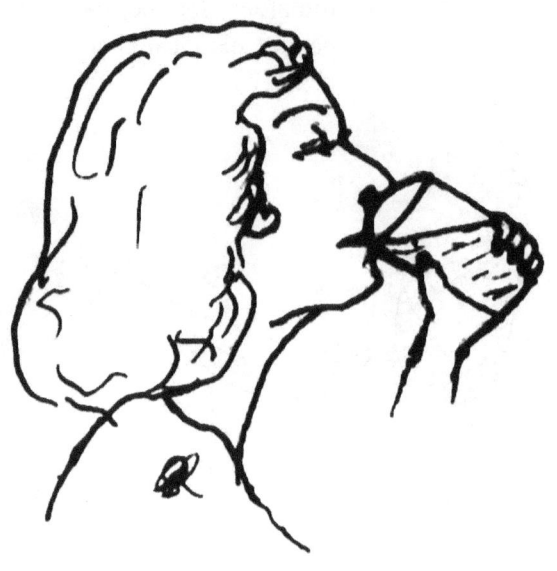

CHAPTER 4

GUIDELINES ON EATING

The following guidelines and menu suggestions have been used by the author to maintain and lose weight when necessary and at the same time supply and adequate amount of energy to be physically active. The daily food intake has been placed in four categories, viz., pre-breakfast, breakfast, lunch, and supper.

Menu Suggestions

PRE-BREAKFAST

1 glass warm water with the juice of one fresh lime
1 large ripe banana

Pre-breakfast serving must be taken upon getting out of bed and at least 45 minutes before eating breakfast.

BREAKFAST SUGGESTIONS

1

1 small orange
1 bowl unsweetened cooked oats

1 boiled egg
1 slice whole wheat bread

2

½ grapefruit
1 sml bowl unsweetened cornmeal
   porridge
1 slice whole wheat bread

3

1 med bowl fresh fruit salad
Steamed callalloo with cod fish

2-3 fingers boiled green bananas

4

1 glass orange juice
1 med bowl bran or fruit and nut
   cereal
1 small cheese omelet
1 slice whole wheat bread

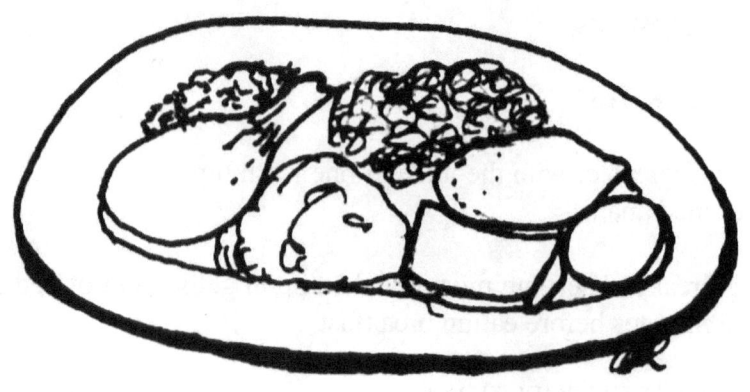

Only liquefied non-dairy milk should be used in porridge or with cereals. Bread should also be eaten unbuttered.

LUNCH

It is advisable to eat your heavy meal around the middle of the day as this meal contains the greatest amounts of calories of all the meals. This practice will avoid unnecessary weight gain as excess calories taken in will have time to be used up in the afternoon. This is not so if taken only a couple hours before retiring to bed.

1
½ chicken breast (baked-b-que)
1 whole wheat dumpling
1 piece pumpkin
¼ cup cooked lentils
1 piece yarn
1 piece sweet potato
1 serving steamed vegetables
1 med bowl toss salad
½ tsp safe salad dressing (ssd)

2
¾ lb steamed fish
1 cup cooked seasoned brown rice
1 piece pumpkin
1 ear boiled corn
1 piece sweet potato
¼ cup split peas
med bowl salad
½ tsp ssd

2
1 serving ALL IN ONE meal
1 bowl salad

4
3 meat balls (vegetable meat)
1 cup ground yam salad
½ baked plantain
1 piece baked sweet potato
1 bowl toss salad

Baked items may be substituted by roasted breadfruit, boiled items, by boiled breadfruit.

Attempt to eliminate white flour products
Substitute with whole wheat, bran and or grain
This helps many lose inches from their guts
So longer lasting energy is what they will gain

SUPPER

1

10-12 whole wheat crackers
1 large mango

2

1 bowl tropical fruit salad (freshly made)

2

1 bowl fruit and nut cereal
1 glass non-dairy milk

4

1 slice special cornmeal or sweet potato
pudding
1 cup unsweetened warm non-dairy milk
(2 tsp. milo may be added)

The above supper suggestions vary in the amounts of calories they supply. No suggestions therefore should be used daily. Each individual must judge for himself or herself whether he wants to gain weight, maintain weight or lose weight. The persons who wish to gain weight may increase the portions of ground food intake or supper proportions. Those who desire to lose weight should decrease the amounts taken. Supper should be taken at least three hours before retiring to bed.

Occasional cleansing
May be mending
Not for abusing
Or you'll be accusing

CHAPTER 5

CLEANSING AND EATING RIGHT

Over years of incorrect eating, our systems tend to become clogged up and function less efficiently. It is strongly recommended therefore that the body undergoes a cleansing process before the implementation of the program. This will facilitate effective absorption of the correctly balanced nutrients by the intestines.

It is best to start the cleansing program on the weekend as you will need ready access to the toilet.

N.B. Before starting any diet or exercise program, it is strongly recommended that you be examined and advised by a physician.

This program tries to utilize products that are readily available at your supermarket or local pharmacy.

First Morning

Simmer 3 teaspoon of Benjamin's herb mixture in half a cup of water. Strain and drink sweetened or unsweetened, first thing in the morning You may substitute the herb mixture with two tea bags of Smooth Move ( ) steeped in 8 ounces of water. Usually, may be found in the health food section of your local grocery store.

Drink one glass of water every half hour for two hours.

Juice 4 grapefruits, 4 oranges, 4 limes and increase the mixture by another one-third of its volume by adding water. Drink one glass every half hour.
Administer an enema in the evening, made up of 1 quart of tepid water and the juice of one lime, strained. An enema bag should be available at your local pharmacy.

UTILIZE LOCAL ITEMS

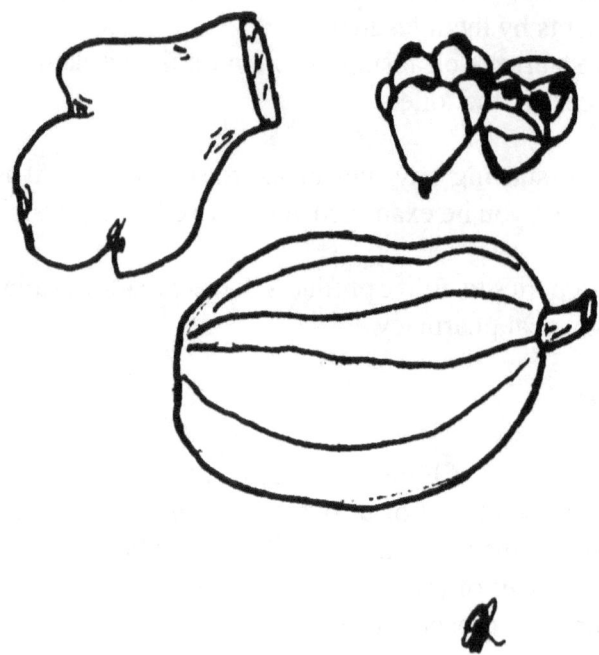

Second Morning

Mix one small packet (approximately 3 teaspoon) of Epson salt in eight ounces of water. Divide in two parts. Drink the first portion followed by eight ounces of water. Drink the second portion half hour later, followed by eight ounces of water. This may again be substituted by two tea bags of Smooth move soaked in eight ounces of water.

Again, this may be substituted by two bags of Smooth Move senna herbal laxative or other similar herbal laxative, steeped in eight ounces water.

Repeat the juice mixture used on the first day, drinking eight ounces every half an hour.

Administer another lime water enema in the evening.

Third Morning

Blend 1 lb. carrots, ½ lb. beet, ½ lb. cho cho or squash, 1 lb. string beans, 1 bundle callalloo or spinach, ½ lb. celery, ½ lb. cauliflower and ½ lb. broccoli.

Start combining the first two items with eight ounces of water, use the resulting juice when strained, to blend the new batch, adding a small amount of water as you progress with your additions. You should try to obtain 12 to 14 glasses of juice.

Drink one glass every half hour to one hour. You may start eating in the evening. Your meal should consist of steamed fish and vegetables.

Subsequent Days

Drink one cup warm water with half a lime squeezed in it. Follow by one ripe banana.

Cook oatmeal for three minutes or less. You may add raisins that have been scalded with boiling water and drained and/or some non-dairy milk. A slice or two of brown toast is optional. Cornmeal porridge may be substituted for the oatmeal. Occasional boiled eggs, steamed callalloo, spinach, or cod fish may be added.

You may have your heavy meal in the middle of the day. This should consist of peas and beans, chicken or fish and four small sized portions of staples chosen from the following foods or from any of the menu suggestions given in the previous chapter.

Half a cup of cooked brown rice, pumpkin, yam, dasheen, breadfruit, plantain, potatoes, sweet potatoes and green banana. A medium sized bowl of fresh chopped green vegetables, such as lettuce, broccoli, and shredded carrots should be included in your meal.

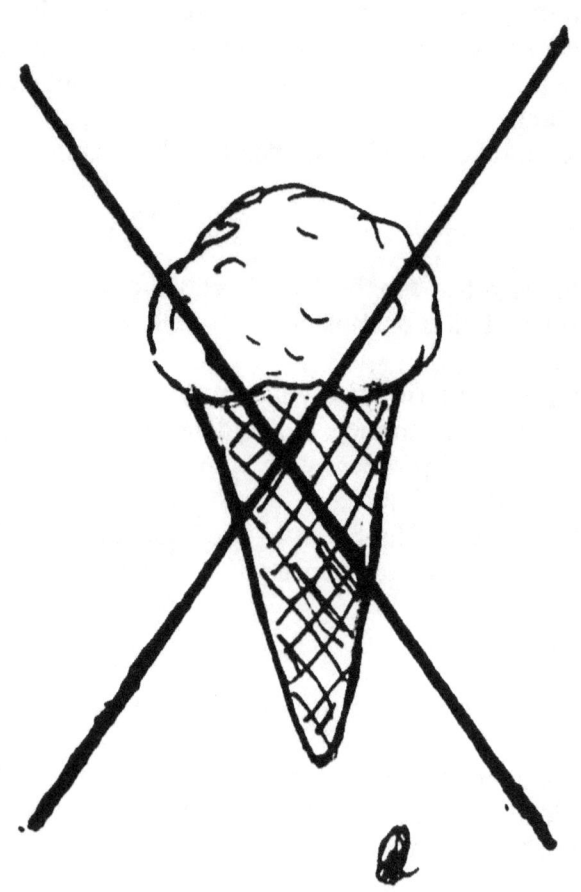

Evening meal may consist of two slices of whole wheat bread or whole wheat biscuits and fresh fruit or fruit salad.

Fruits may be eaten throughout the day as snack.

Drinks should include 6-8 glasses of water daily and natural vegetable and /or fruit juices without sugar.

Foods to Avoid

Cakes, sweet biscuits, white flour products, sweets, fried foods, ice cream, pasta, red meats, coffee, black tea.

You should record your weight prior to starting this program. It will not be necessary for you to weigh more often than once per week as weight loss should not be more than one to two pounds per week. A more rapid weight loss is an indication of the need to increase your food intake.

Persons with chronic illnesses should eliminate or reduce their intake of salt, margarine, oil and seasonings or apices.

N.B.: This program has not been scientifically tested but has been used successfully by the author and others, with no major side effects. Gripes may be experienced on the cleansing days. It is therefore necessary to maintain the high fluid intake recommended to help alleviate these symptoms, should they occur. Should you experience severe pain or fainting, call 911, (119 in Jamaica, W.I.) and contact your physician immediately, and go to the emergency room.

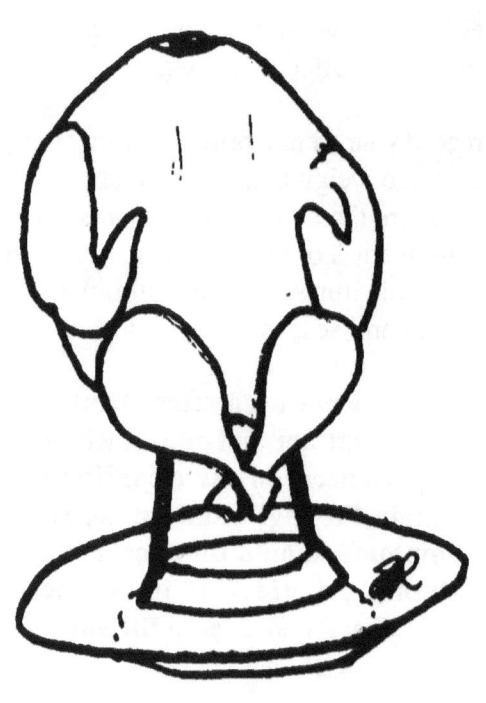

CHAPTER 6

RECIPES

BAKED-B-QUED CHICKEN
1 lb. chicken breast or other desired chicken part
Dash black pepper
1 stalk scallion or celery
1 twig thyme
½ scotch bonnet pepper (seed removed)
Dash salt
1 onion

Method
Preheat oven to 350F. Cut chicken in desired sizes. Season with black pepper, salt, chopped scallion or celery, onion and thyme. Let soak for twenty minutes. Place seasoned chicken in baking tin, cover with foil and place on preheated oven for 30 minutes. Use brush to put sauce on chicken. Replace in oven for another 15 minutes without covering. Turn chicken over and brush the other side with the sauce. Replace in oven for another 15 minutes or until cooked. Serves 2 persons.

Sauce
¼ cup tomato ketchup
1 tbsp sugar
1 peg ginger
½ tsp corn flour
1 peg garlic
¼ cup water
1/8 cup vinegar

This guide can lead to no extra cost
As your desire for unhealthy food is lost
You find yourself buying healthier foods
And making your meals from your home stored goods

Method

Scrape, wash and crush ginger and garlic. Place in sauce pan. Add all other ingredients. Mix together until corn flour blends in. Simmer for 5 minutes.

VEGE-MEAT BALLS
½ cup vegetable-mince or any other ground vegetable mince
1 egg, beaten
Black pepper
Salt
1 onion, diced
1 stalk scallion or celery, diced
1 tbsp soy sauce
3 level tbsp flour
Coconut or olive oil

Method

Soak vegetable mince in hot water for 15 minutes. Drain them and set aside. Add seasoning and soy sauce to beaten egg. Add this mixture to drained vegetable-mince. Mix thoroughly, then add flour and continue to mix.

Heat a small sauce pan. Use adequate amount of oil for frying. When oil is hot, use spoon to form small balls of vegetable mixture. Drop in sauce pan and remove as soon as crisp brown. Place on paper towel.

SAFE SALAD DRESSING
1tsp olive oil or coconut oil
1/8 cup vinegar
2 tsp sugar

Method

Place all ingredients in a jar. Cover and shake well.

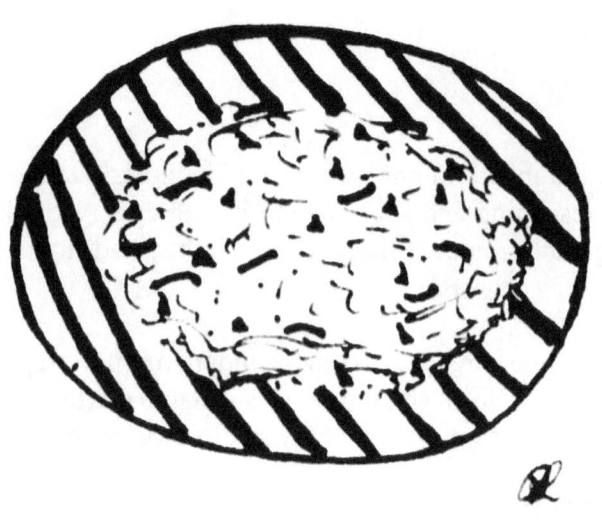

SEASONED BROWN RICE
2 cups water
1 cup brown rice
1 pack chicken noodle soup

Method
Bring water to boil, then add chicken noodle. Lower heat and let boil for a further 3 minutes. Add rice that has been washed and drained. Further lower heat. Cover pot and let simmer. Add 2 tsp margarine when water is no longer above the rice. Mix in with a fork. Cover until rice is cooked.

ALL IN ONE
1 med sized dried coconut (grated and juiced in 3 cups water)
4 slices green breadfruit, peeled
4 slices yam
4 slices dasheen or one medium size sweet potato
½ lb. cod fish (soaked overnight in water and drained)
½ lb. chicken (cut in serving pieces and seasoned)
3 stalks scallion or celery
2 twigs thyme
1 scotch bonnet pepper (deseeded and dices)
1 large onion
Salt to taste

Method
Bring coconut juice to boil. Reduce heat to medium. Add deboned fish and chicken pieces. Add potato, dasheen or sweet potato, yam, and breadfruit. Do not allow liquid to dry out. You may reduce the heat or add small amounts of hot water. Add seasoning and salt to taste.

Planting a back door garden is an inexpensive way to go
With two beans from your pantry, hundreds will grow
Remember to water after you sow
And when you reap you will be able to stow

FRESH TROPICAL FRUIT SALAD
1 pineapple
2 lbs. watermelon
2 small paw paw or papaya
1 large mango
3 large bananas
3 oranges
Juice of 1 lime, strained
1 tablespoon strawberry syrup

Method
Peel and dice pineapple, watermelon, paw paw or papaya, mango and bananas and place in a large bowl. Peel oranges deep enough to expose the pulp all around. Use a sharp knife to remove the pulp in peg-like portions.

Mix the juice of 1 lime with tablespoon syrup. Pour this over the combination of fruits. Chill and serve.

SPECIAL CORNMEAL PUDDING
½ medium sized coconut, grated and 2 cups mild expressed
1 tbsp flour
2 cups refined cornmeal
1/3 cup brown sugar
2 tsp vanilla
½ tsp nutmeg
1 tsp cinnamon
½ tsp salt
½ cup raisins
1 tbsp butter

Method
Mix all ingredients, excepting cornmeal, together and bring to boil. Mix cornmeal in 2 cups water and add to liquid mixture, stirring constantly. Lower heat and continue stirring for 7 minutes. Pour mixture into greatest baking tin and bake for 15 minutes in oven, preheated to 350F. Serve hot or cold.

SPECIAL SWEET POTATO PUDDING
1 medium sized coconut, grated and 3 cups milk expressed (coconut may be substituted with one can coconut milk diluted as appropriate)
2 lbs. sweet potato, grated
½ cup brown sugar
1 tsp powdered ginger
2 tsp vanilla
½ tsp nutmeg
1 tsp cinnamon

The deserts in this guide include sugar for beginner's taste
But do make an effort to decrease that to half in this case
If weight loss is your goal, do this in haste
And you will be successful as if winning a race

¾ cup raisins
1 ½ cups hot water
1 tbsp flour
1 tbsp margarine
1 tsp salt

Method
Mix all ingredients together, excepting grated potato. When the mixture has been totally blended, add potato and continue to mix. Pour into greased baking tin and place in oven that has been preheated to 375F. Let bake for approximately one hour. Reduce temperature to 300F for 15 minutes.

SWEET POTATO SALAD
2 lbs. sweet potato, peeled, diced and boiled
2 tsp mayonnaise
1 egg, boiled, stripped, and diced
½ cup split beans, boiled
1 onion, diced
1 cup whole kernel corn.
Black pepper
Salt
Garlic powder

Remember your juices are important
Eliminate the sugar if you can
Substitute guava sometimes
And for a tangy taste, use limes

Method
Mix all cooked ingredients together. Add salt, garlic powder and pepper to taste. Sprinkle with parsley.

Sweet potato may be substituted by any kind of yam, breadfruit, or irish potato.

JUNE PLUM DRINK
3 green june plums, peeled
2 limes, juiced
3 tablespoons sugar
2 quarts water

Method
Blend slices of june plum in 1 quart water. Strain and add juice of limes and rounded tablespoons sugar. Add remaining water. Serve with ice.

PAWRANGE DRINK
2 small paw paws or papayas, deseeded and peeled
4 large oranges, juiced
2 cups water
1 rounded tbsp sugar
1 lime, juiced

Method
Blend paw paw or papaya in water. Add orange juice, lime juice and sugar and blend for one minute. Serve with ice.

Don't be confused with the different terms that are used
For example, vege-meat is similar to tofu
However, limit your substitution, so this guide is not abused
So success will be for all and not just for a few

MINCE A LA POTATO
½ cup vegetable-mince
1 large irish potato, diced and cooked
1 small can whole kernel corn
½ tsp salt
Black pepper
Garlic powder
2 tbsp ketchup
1 tsp margarine
1 onion, diced
1 stalk scallion or celery
½ scotch bonnet pepper, deseeded and diced.

Method
Soak vegetable-mince in hot water for 15 minutes, the drain. Place margarine in sauce pan until melted. Add onion, scallion, pepper and sauce on low heat for 5 minutes. Add remaining ingredients. Cover and let simmer on low heat for another 10 minutes. Do not allow to dry out. You may add a few tablespoons of water.

VEGE-STEAK A LA POTATO
1 cup vegetable steak
1 large irish potato, peeled and diced.
1 can butter beans
½ tsp salt
Dash black pepper
1 tsp garlic powder
2 tbsp soy sauce
1 onion diced
2 tbsp coconut oil
½ scotch bonnet pepper, deseeded and diced

No one can say
He won't die on day
But why not stay
For as long as you may

Method

Soak vegetable steak in hot water for 10 minutes, then drain and season with salt, pepper, garlic powder and soy sauce. Place oil in skillet and heat. Place vegetable steak in hot oil and brown on both sides. Add diced potato and onion. Cover and let simmer on low heat until potatoes are cooked. Add butter beans and simmer for another three minutes. Serve hot.

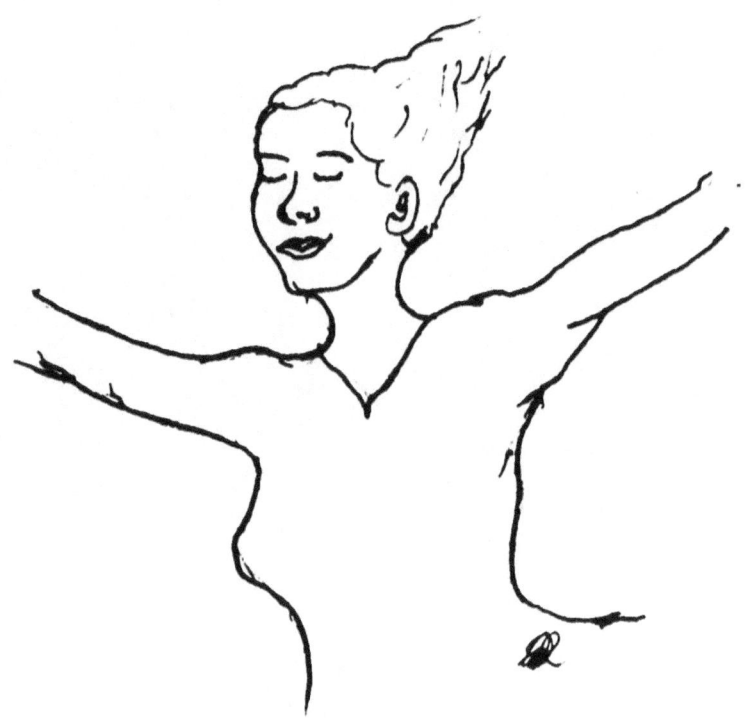

I FEEL GOOD!!

PART II

CHAPTER 7

THE EXPERIENCES

The untimely and unexpected passing of the late editor Dr. Lorna Nembhard created a void in my dreams for this book resulting in doubts in proceeding with the publishing of the book. She had created so much of the spirit of this book through her belief that this book was one that could be valuable to those who could not afford to purchase or follow expensive weight loss programs, and therefore it was worth publishing. It was her spirit of enthusiasm, and her belief in the simplicity of the design of this book that was the driving force for completing this short, and easy to read manual. For years, I believed the idea of using this written piece to guide and instruct others, had passed with her passing. This unpublished piece was locked away for many years, actually forgotten as the hope of it being a helpful health guide to all, regardless of the level of intellect, faded.

Today, as I proceed with post graduate studies, I have come to realize that no information that is valuable to health is useless, especially when the implications of following this guide can only be positive. In addition, no instruction locked away in a cupboard can have any impact at all. Moreover, at a time when the drastic effects of the present economical status have impacted so many persons across the globe in a negative way, choosing an expensive weight control program becomes very low on the priority list. In reviewing this guide, I became more convinced that now, more than at any other time, many people could benefit by simply choosing foods, and other items from their regular grocery basket with the purchase of perhaps one or two items not usually included in the regular grocery list.

At this point, it is appropriate to welcome our new editor, Dr. Prudencia Reid-Kintaudi who has approached this creation with the same energy and optimism as our late editor Dr. Lorna Nembhard did. In proceeding, I will trace the benefits I have experienced from adhering to guidelines of this book, and also the symptoms I suffered when I diverted from the guidelines for an extended period.

Both Dr. Reid-Kintaudi and I believe that with the rising economic deficits seen throughout world economies, there is less money available for healthcare, and in particular, Primary Healthcare which emphasizes *prevention*.

How often have you gone to a doctor, especially in the United States, where I presently live, and hear the importance of changing one's diet to a healthy diet that will prevent the diseases of the affluent people who live a sedentary lifestyle? It is significant to note that these diseases, once labeled "diseases of the affluent," no longer discriminate, but are regularly seen across all sectors of society. They ultimately lead to visits to the doctor, as resulting unpleasant symptoms persists.

More often than not, you will be given medication to treat whatever complaint you have, and upon your return visit, you may receive additional medication to counteract the side effects of the medication you were given for your initial complaint at your first visit to the doctor. Ultimately, the saga continues until you find yourself taking numerous different medications to combat various different signs, and symptoms. My bet is that up to this point, you have not been educated on a healthy lifestyle, including diet, and exercise.

I must admit that for numerous years, I found pleasure in unhealthy eating. One of my favorite hobbies was baking Jamaican Christmas puddings.

It did not have to be Christmas to find an excuse to bake this rich, wine, and rum soaked pudding. Birthdays were an excuse to bake these puddings that we often referred to as fruit cake, in its slightly drier form. Special dinner occasions, and weddings were other excuses. I eagerly looked forward to attending weddings because there, one could get some of the richest, rum soaked puddings, otherwise known as wedding cakes. Although this was usually rationed, mainly because of the great expense in preparing this delicacy, I found myself scheming about how to get more than one piece of this precious ration. Nevertheless, there was no rationing of this precious commodity after I became an adult, so at Christmas time, I ate to my heart's content. Actually, I ate Christmas pudding until I became ill. Following three days of binging on this product, I became so nauseated, and noted that my blood pressure was increased, and that if I did not stop eating this I would die. My normal blood pressure was usually 90/60, a level that would probably be considered too low for many persons. Each time I would visit the doctor, after making myself sick, I would register a blood pressure reading of 120/80, which the doctor would say was normal. There was no way of convincing any of the doctors that this reading was simply too high for me, and that it was causing me to have severe headaches. I had to learn therefore to stop eating the wrong foods, do a cleansing, and resume my exercise program.

Christmas pudding was not the adversary. Rather, it was my binging on Christmas pudding that was my adversary. There were periods in my life when I binged on extremely fatty foods, fast foods, chocolates, and other sweets. I found it very difficult, to almost impossible to walk away from a buffet luncheon, or dinner without sampling all the deserts present there.

Controlling a stable weight became a problem. My body weight fluctuated between 138 and 148 pounds, stabilizing more often at 145 pounds.

Something significant was taking place. I noticed that when I was between 145 pounds and 148 pounds, my blood pressure reached 120/80, and even rose to 125/95, accompanied by severe headaches. Knowing the pattern of these headaches, that would not ease with pain medication, I was forced to try bringing my weight back to under 145 pounds. I know that many of you reading this guide can guess that this task would be a difficult one.

Being faced with the possibility of having a stroke, and being disabled, with so many persons depending on me for one reason or the other, I was able to muster up the discipline to eat healthily for a while.

I was on a yo-yo, or roller coaster lifestyle. When my body weight was below 145 pounds, my blood pressure was at an acceptable level that caused me no headaches. Above that body weight, it was at the normally accepted 120/80 which not only caused me severe headaches, but also was not high enough for the doctor to treat me with anti-hypertensive medication. My lifestyle was out of control. I worked hard all my life; did not get enough sleep; and did no form of exercises for long periods. My clothes didn't fit right anymore when I was 148 pounds. I did not want to put on tennis outfits to play my favorite game because my thighs were too big, and filled with cellulite. My self-esteem was damaged, and I felt trapped in a box.

I had to do something. With these headaches, and all the stress that had complicated my life (which would take another encyclopedia sized manuscript to explain), I needed to start out slowly. Although I hated walking, starting to walk one mile, for three consecutive days, made the intensity of the headaches subside.

Thereafter, I felt more confident, or rather, less fearful of having drastic, unhealthy experiences, and was then able to tolerate more physical exertion. I would start running, in a slow trot for about half a mile for the next two days and increase to a mile. At no time did I overexert myself. It was important for me to feel safe if I wanted to benefit from this program.

An integral part of my health program was to drink six to eight glasses of water each day. Initially, drinking water was a difficult task. I just needed something to change the taste of the water, which was just too bland. At first I had to add a syrup, just enough to give a touch of sweetness. Later, I could drink the water with a teaspoon of lemon juice for each glass of water. However, I noted that despite the healthy lifestyle I had now adopted, I began to have pains in my low back, radiating down both lower limbs. These symptoms became more and more intense, resulting in sleep disturbances. They progressed to the point where it was difficult to stand, and later to sit. I had never heard of chemical sciatica until I attended a medical symposium in Kingston, Jamaica. Physical therapists were privileged to present one paper at this symposium which featured mainly doctors. During the physical therapy presentation, back pain and sciatica were discussed in details, with a brief sentence on chemically-induced back ache and sciatica.

As strange as this sounded, it started to make sense to me. You see, I had been thoroughly tested, with no significant findings that could explain my symptoms.

There was one problem. I could find little to no study on chemical-induced backache and sciatica. Searching the internet produced a short paragraph describing the possible distribution of the pain, and nothing on the possible cause. During the time period that I suffered these sciatica-like pains, there was as not much information on the internet as we have today. However, having recently surfed the web again, I have found that there is still not much more enlightenment on this subject. The partial discovery, and I say partial, because my case study was incomplete as I did not have the financing to eliminate the elements in the substances that would be implicated as the root cause of my ailment, was a miracle. It was sheer serendipity that my sister-in-law encouraged me to visit a doctor in California and be properly tested, since all tests done in Jamaica were fruitless in identifying a cause for my pains. It took over a week to arrange for a complete physical to be done. However, just before initiating these tests, I noticed that I had no pains. I knew it had to be something I was ingesting in Jamaica that I was not ingesting in California. We set out to isolate every item I had put in my mouth since being in California and analyzed, and compared them with what I was eating in Jamaica. The thought that the cause of my ailments could be in the atmosphere was also considered. This idea complicated things a bit, since we thought atmospheric testing of samples on air in California, and in Jamaica would entail expensive chemical tests which we were just not able to entertain at this difficult, and challenging period of my life. Hence the process of elimination began.

It did not take very long to come to a conclusion. The food intake in my daily diet in Jamaica was very much similar to my diet in California. The most striking difference was the fact that in Jamaica I drank chlorine-treated potable water, while in California, I drank bottled spring water. I immediately cancelled all plans to have a thorough medical examination done and returned home to Jamaica. Then the experiments started. I would go back to drinking chlorinated potable water for two weeks in Jamaica, and the excruciating back and leg pains would begin. I would drink only spring water for two weeks, using it to make all my teas and other beverages, and my back and leg pains would go. My body had become so sensitive to whatever element was in the chlorinated potable water that if I even had two beverages, mixed with ice from regular tap water, the pains would increase to an intolerable level.

Please bear in mind that chlorine has not been implicated as the element identified as the causative agent in my dilemma. The term "chlorinated potable water," has only been used to identify the source containing the causative agent for my pains. I had tried to get further investigations, or studies done in this area.

I went as far as giving an informal study I conducted with a few of my physical therapy patients who suffered similar symptoms as I did, to the then head of a university's community health faculty, with a request for an expansion of this study.

I was rightfully advised that numerous studies needed to be conducted into the elements contained in the chlorinated potable water in Jamaica. I am still hoping that this study will be revived and expanded, since my initial study included all the patients, who complained of back pain with sciatica-like symptoms; who had been extensively tested; and who could not find a cause for their pains; being a small population of five persons.

I remember some of these patients having extreme tenderness of the soft tissues across the low back, buttocks, and thighs. Though my study was possibly filled with biases, particularly because of the lack of truly controlled empirical studies, the informal qualitative examination gave me an idea of what was happening, and whether elimination of chlorinated potable water correlated with a reduction in symptoms. On all the cases examined, a positive response was obtained, whenever there was an adherence to guidelines. My informal questionnaire was very simple and included such questions as:

1) How strong is your back and leg pain today? Give a rating.
2) Did you use bottled spring water for every liquid you drank this week?
3) Did you have significant pain during the week?
4) What was the brand of the bottled water you drank this week?
5) Did you do the prescribed exercises and activities given in this clinic?

In each case the symptoms were significantly decreased when the patient adhered to the use of the bottled water regime.

In my case, not all bottled water could be correlated with the decrease or resolution of my back and leg pains. There were some quite expensive bottled water that were imported into Jamaica, that I correlated with my increase back and leg pains. An examination of the elements written on those bottled waters, identified chlorine, sodium, calcium, and other substances. I was however, able to ingest calcium in the tablet form, and sodium in table salt without any adverse effects, as long as I adhered to the trusted bottled spring water regime, but it had to be spring water that did not have any of the above elements. After a while, I learned to tell the difference in the taste of the different brands of spring water. I knew that if one brand tasted similar to regular potable tap water in Jamaica, then it must have the elements added to it or it was tap water being disguised as spring water. I soon learned to rely on only two brands of spring water sold in Jamaica. There may have been other reliable brands, but once I had isolated two brands, I decided to stick with what I knew. This practice has worked well for me over the past ten years, to the point where I am now comfortably able to drink regular potable water, or beverage processed with chlorinated potable water, for a day or two without any of the former side effects I once suffered. This did not happen overnight. It appeared as if my body needed to have years of cleansing from the harmful elements. For the past year or two, I have had little recurrence of my back and leg pains. If minor symptoms occur, they usually last one day, and are usually a result of diverging from my strict water regime for more than two days.

CHAPTER 8

WHAT IS HAPPENING TODAY

Today, at 55 years old, I am a picture of health. I avoid red meats, too many sweets, too many white flour products, and too much oily foods. I bake, grill or steam most of my meats. Except for escovitch fish, I seldom ever fry my meats.

I drink 16 ounces of warm water with a teaspoon of lemon or lime juice on waking up in the mornings. This is followed by eating one large ripe banana. This regime regularized my bowels and avoided the once problematic constipation from which I suffered. I try to follow up my first water intake with at least three more bottles of water for the day. My desire is to drink the desired six to eight 8 oz bottles of water each day.

Rest and regular exercise are very vital to optimal performance of the human body. I just do not feel well when I lack exercise or sleep. I have a rigorous schedule which involves, doing home health physical therapy at least 25 hours per week, managing one of my husband's dental clinics another 30 hours per week, and school work for another 35 hours per week. This does not leave much time for household activities, or for sleeping. I manage to carve out three 30 to 60 minute exercise sessions each week, mainly done indoors. This is obviously unsatisfactory for me, since I prefer one form of recreation that relieves all my emotional, mental, and physical stress. I would do anything to have a regular tennis partner who lives in my housing subdivision and is available two nights per week. My experience is that I am a renewed, spirited individual after an hour of hard hitting singles tennis. Another form of recreation for me is swimming in the sea. It provides a form of all-body activity with similar benefits to that of playing tennis, but for me the joy of the competitiveness in playing tennis provides greater emotional release. This is why living in Jamaica, for me, creates the opportunity for a healthier lifestyle within the scope of my affordability.

Notwithstanding, I am therefore striving to manage my time in a more efficient manner that will afford me an average of seven hours sleep each night, while living in America.

I have been asked about the effects of menopause on my body. Ironically, I started to have brief episodes of heat especially at 4 or 5 a.m. when I really wanted to sleep since I stay up very late. I quickly learned to keep a glass of water by my bedside and drink it as soon as I was awaken by the heat and nausea. After approximately one year of this practice, the symptoms of menopause practically disappeared, or were so negligible that they were hardly noticed. If I failed to drink a glass of water when these symptoms started, then they would persist until I did so.

I do not expect that this is the panacea for all women who experience severe symptoms of menopause, but I think if it worked for me, it may also work for other women. Each woman has to evaluate herself and take the necessary ameliorating steps for attaining a level of comfort with regards to menopause, and the menopausal symptoms.

I have also been asked about minerals and vitamin supplements. At present, I take one or two regular multivitamin tablets each day. This is not a rigid practice as I have gone for a few days on occasion without access to vitamins when I travel away from home. There was a time when I regularly took calcium tablets, and other cartilage building supplements on a daily basis. My reaction to these additives were the opposite of what was expected. At my age, calcium supplements and cartilage building supplements have been recommended, but unfortunately after two weeks of taking them, I start having pains in my knee joints; sometimes extending to other joints. My recent bone density scan showed that I was still in the normal acceptable range. I try instead to eat lots of fruits and vegetables that are high in the minerals and vitamins that the body needs. I cannot determine if there is any relationship to my recurring knee pains and my taking of these supplements. Again each individual has to decide along with his or her personal physician, what is best practice for that person.

I would like to offer a few words of comfort and encouragement to those persons who have difficulty adhering to a healthy lifestyle. This is not an easy feat, especially when diverting from any guide to healthy living produces a sense of failure.

I would say to anyone who has failed on occasions, "Never give up." It is the persistence in resuming after every failure, that eventually builds the self control to maintain a healthy lifestyle. Like many individuals who fail at adhering to a program of healthy living, it was very difficult initially for me to follow my own guideline for healthy living, despite the fact that I felt healthier when I actually adhered to the guidelines of this book. You should keep in mind that novel practices are difficult to comply with initially, but that resuming the program after each derailment, builds the strength to adhere for longer periods each time. As your body gets used to the new way of eating and living, you should develop the desire to maintain a healthy lifestyle. I think most of us are happy that scientists like William Gilbert and Ben Franklin did not give up after their first failure. Otherwise we may still be in the "dark" today; no electric bulbs from which to get light to read; no computers to send e-mail messages, twits, blogs, etc.

CHAPTER 9

WHO IS THE TRUE AUTHOR?

I often ponder about my life experiences, making sure never to lament about the things that could have been interpreted as disasters, but rather to look at them as challenges that bring a sense of achievement when they are controlled.

One thing that has caused me to ponder on the events of my life and the opportune time at which they occur, is the knowledge that comes to me through my own experiences, that forces me to look at solutions to the problems. In finding solutions to my own problems, usually others are relieved of their problems also.

I ask myself questions like, "Why did patients having similar experiences with back pain come to my clinic at the time I was also having back and leg pains?" or "Why did I know certain things were going to happen before they did?" In addition, I have seen too many miracles that cannot be explained as mere accidents, or coincidences; too many words of knowledge that came to me out of nowhere, or as confirmation while meditating on my Divine Power, the Almighty God, to ignore the fact that He had everything to do with the writing of this book.

I chose therefore to close this book with a prayer of thanksgiving.

Almighty Father, maker of heaven and earth
I give you thanks for the experiences and inspiration
that led to the writing of this guide to health.
I pray that the wisdom imparted in this creation
will not only bring health, but also wealth
to all who seek understanding from the notion
that you give wisdom, and knowledge, health,
and strength and know all that man needs is devotion

to practice your laws of love, and heart felt
caring for your perfect universal, geometrical creation,
without selfish greed, or desire to control all the wealth
which is sufficient for each man to have his portion,
to endue him with perfect, enduring strength.
Thank you that this guide will help many in this nation
who normally could not afford to access guides to good health,
and for its success across the globe in this era of globalization.

REFERENCES

Centers for Disease Control and Prevention (2009). U.S. Department of Health and Human Services. *http://www.cdc.gov/NCCdphp/ publications/AAG/obesity.htm*

Centers for Disease Control and Prevention (2009). U.S. Department of Health and Human Services. *http://www.cdc.gov/stroke/ stroke_facts.htm*

Cleveland Clinic (2009). Number one in heart care for 15 years. *http:// my.clevelandclinic.org/heart/women/teenhealth/typesoffats.aspx*

Office of the Surgeon General (2007). U.S. Department of Health and Human Services. *http://www.surgeongeneral.gov/topics/obesity/ calltoaction/fact_consequences. htm*

Master of Public Health Program (1996) Synopsis of lectures in epidemiology and nutrition. Department of Social and Preventive Medicine, University of the West Indies, Mona Campus, Jamaica W.I.

Sinha, D.P (1996) Food, Nutrition and Health in the Caribbean. Caribbean Food and Nutrition Institute, Kingston, Jamaica W. I., pp. 10-49.

GLOSSARY

Coconut-   Culturally in Jamaica where this book was
                                initially conceived, it is the practice to
                                grate the fruit of the coconut and extract
                                the juice by hand. However, this may be
                                substituted by using a can of coconut milk
                                obtained from your grocery store and
                                diluted with water to achieve the desired
                                amount.

Dasheen, yam, sweet potato, cassava, yuca—perennial herbaceous starchy
                                vines; grown mainly in Africa, Caribbean,
                                Asia, Latin America, and Oceania (*http://
                                en.wikipedia.org*). These may substitute
                                each other in the menus given

Scallion—   commonly known in the Caribbean as
                                escallion.

June plum—   popular fruit in Jamaica. This may be
                                substituted with American plum.

Vege-mince—   A brand of meat substitute made of
                                vegetables, minced and dried, often sold
                                in Jamaica and other Caribbean islands.

www.ingramcontent.com/pod-product-compliance
Lightning Source LLC
Chambersburg PA
CBHW031302280526
45784CB00004B/1958